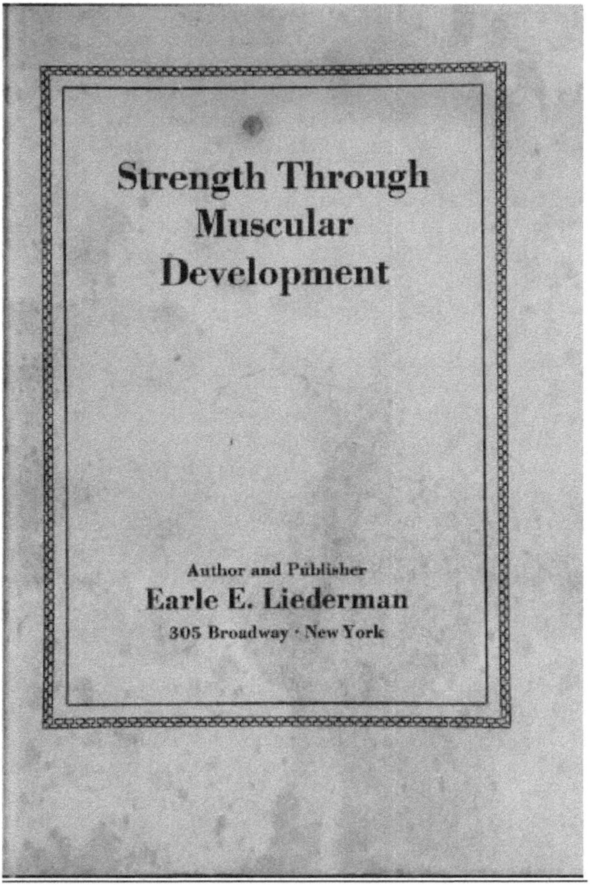

# Strength Through Muscular Development

Author and Publisher
## Earle E. Liederman
305 Broadway · New York

# STRENGTH THROUGH MUSCULAR DEVELOPMENT

(ORIGINAL VERSION, RESTORED)

By

## EARLE LIEDERMAN

Original Publisher: Earle Liederman, 305 Broadway, New York, 1927

PUBLISHED BY O'Faolain Patriot LLC, Copyright 2011

info@PhysicalCultureBooks.com

ISBN-13: 978-1467976626

ISBN-10: 1467976628

Published in the United States of America

To Order More Copies Visit: Physical Culture Books.com

# STRENGTH THROUGH MUSCULAR DEVELOPMENT

A boy who enters school at eight years and graduates at eighteen, has during that ten years given up at least six hours a day to exercising and cultivating his mind. There was a time when those who run the schools gave no thought whatever to the cultivation of the body, but during the last generation the necessity of physical exercise has been recognized, and today the heads of schools see to it that their pupils are compelled to take part in sports, games and exercises which make for bodily betterment.

Undeniably, the brain can stand more work than the body can. A student can spend four hours in the class room and four more in concentrated study, without becoming brain-tired; in fact, his mental powers are developed by such application. The same student could not spend eight hours per day at equally hard physical work without becoming exhausted. Two hours of vigorous play every day is sufficient to promote healthy bodily growth in a schoolboy, while half of that is plenty enough to keep a college student in condition.

But play—athletic sports and games—admirable as they are, are neither the only nor the best means of physical education. Especially is this true at institutions where sport is systematized, and the big teams get most of the attention. For there the weak boy or youth, the one who most needs the exercise and the physical training, has to step aside and make room for the other boy who is already so good that his presence on the playing field is an asset to the institution.

At many colleges and schools, physical drill is required; but the very fact that it is compulsory robs it of much of the value. "Setting up" exercises are better than nothing, but when performed under compulsion and in a haphazard way by a large group they tend to become a monotonous hardship instead of an invigorating pastime.

Little or no effort is made to explain to the individual student his own capacities for bodily improvement, nor to awaken in him the desire for physical perfection.

For those who are interested in some particular sport, every facility is provided. High-salaried coaches will teach him all they know about how to play some game, and his hours for study will be arranged so as not to interfere with his hours for game practice. Members of teams are given special privileges. Under this system all that is required of the non-athletic student is that he shall appear regularly in the cheering section.

Anyone interested in the physical betterment of the rising generation cannot help being struck with the popularity of the playground as compared with the unpopularity of the gymnasium. The only time most students voluntarily go to the gym is when there is a chance to see a basketball game, or a boxing or wrestling tournament.

A student cannot graduate from school or college without passing specified tests, and to pass those tests proves that he has more knowledge and brain-power than at the beginning of his school work. I believe that it is possible to devise a system of physical education that will be just as successful in developing the physique of the pupil as the present system improves his mind.

But at present the weak and undeveloped man who wishes to become strong and healthy has to have recourse to the services of private teachers who will give him the kind of individual training his case demands. And such people are legion. Why, I myself in the course of a little over one year, heard from nearly half a million men and boys whose letters proved that they were interested in getting bigger, better and healthier bodies.

I mention that not as an instance of my own popularity, but as evidence of the tremendous and widespread interest in the cultivation of the body. Those letters came from all kinds and classes of citizens, all the way from the middle-aged business men who wished to regain their youthful figures and energy, down to college students and schoolboys who were after results which they could not obtain through the facilities afforded by the physical departments of their own institutions.

It has come to be recognized that systematic physical training will do as much for the body as systematic study will do for the mind. More and more people are becoming interested in acquiring for themselves beautiful, shapely, strong and healthy bodies.

And interest is the secret of development. Any teacher will tell you that a boy will learn vastly more about a subject in which he is interested, than in a subject which bores him. As a teacher of physical culture I can assure you that a man or boy who is interested in seeing how much strength and muscular development he can obtain, will improve in both respects ten times as rapidly as the other individual who looks upon exercise as a necessary nuisance, which must be done for health's sake.

There are many who are what you might call fatalists about their own bodies. They think that development "just happens," that either you have strength, or you haven't and that it is flying in the face of nature to try and increase your own physical assets.

I have in mind two brothers of exactly opposite types, both physically and mentally. The younger of the two, a tall, rangy youth of twenty-one became dissatisfied with what he called his "scrawni- ness" and embarked on a system of home training that called for a half-hour's daily exercise of a rather rigorous character. The older brother, who was also tall but much broader-shouldered and heavier all-around, was inclined to sneer and jibe. He said to me, "I don't care what you say—strength doesn't come that way! Why look at me—when I was a kid I worked every summer on a farm. I would start in at six o'clock in the morning and work until supper time. Nearly twelve hours every day at plowing, reaping, spading, hoeing and all kinds of hard work. No wonder I have big shoulders and a strong back. My arms and legs are not very big, but then I have small bones. I feel that I have as much muscle and strength as nature intends me to have, and I think that Ed is a fool to think he can get even as big as I am by monkeying a little while every day with those Exercisers.' Why, he never did any hard work in all his life. Let him do what I did and he can get strength if he wants it so badly."

Now, happily that younger brother was one of the kind that is not easily discouraged. He just went on quietly at his exercise, studying his weak points, and learning how to build them up. Also he had very definite ideas of just what he wanted to accomplish. For instance, he knew that in order to be well-proportioned he should have a 43-inch chest, and although his chest measured only 36 inches when he started, he knew that it was possible to get a chest as big as he wanted, because he knew of other men who had made that much improvement. To make a long story short, the younger man did get just the development he wanted (and the strength also) and now instead of being known as "the skinny boy" he is known as "that big, finely built boy." In fact, he now exceeds his older brother in development and strength just as much as he was inferior to him a year ago. But then he felt in his heart and soul that it was possible for him to improve. He refused to admit that while other men could build up, he could not. While the

9

older brother who declined to make the effort necessary for improvement, now contents himself by insisting that there was "something unnatural" about Ed's growing so much huskier after he was twenty-one.

While I am on the subject, I can not help saying that I am continually puzzled by the attitude some people have towards strength and development.

Recently I was consulted by a young chap who certainly had nothing to brag about in the way of physical attractions. To begin with he was rather less than average height, and was of the flat-chested, round-shouldered variety. Now from my point of view he was at least twenty-five pounds lighter than he should have been. Evidently he placed a high value on his personal appearance, for he dressed in a way to emphasize what points he had. A good tailor had cut his clothes, and the back of the coat was well-shaped, and in order to make him appear broad-shouldered it was tapered into the waist line and tightly belted. The trousers were rather full at the top of the legs in a way that made it seem as though he had some thigh development; and like many other flat-chested men he had a trick of buttoning only the bottom button of his coat. That made his coat flare open at the top, and thus gave the impression that there was a real chest inside of the coat.

While he was talking to me I noticed that he was looking over me in a disapproving way and he stared so earnestly at my neck that I wondered whether my collar was soiled, or my necktie disarranged. Finally he blurted out, "Mr. Liederman, I do want to get stronger and to have a better figure. But if you take me in hand and train me I want you to promise that you will not make me too big. Now, I wouldn't want to be as broad as you are, and particularly I wouldn't care to have a neck like yours." "Why, what's the matter with my neck?" "Oh," he said, "it is too big. It looks like a wrestler's neck. I don't want to be built like a wrestler or a Hercules. I want to be slim and have a good shape at the same time. I think that if a man has a thick neck and thick wrists he looks coarse, and would be out of place in a fashionable training room. You know, Mr. Liederman, the fashionable trend is toward slender- ness—to keep your boyish figure. The women like a slender, well-made man, but these big truck-horses of men disgust them." Seeing that I am fairly tall and weigh only about 175 pounds I was rather surprised that I should be considered monstrously large, but I controlled myself and said: "Man, I have no intention of giving you what you call a 'truck horse build,' but if I am to give you a real build it will be necessary to make your chest several inches bigger. That means that the upper part of your back will be broader and that your sides will taper in finely from your arm-pits to the sides of your waist. Also your chest will get rounded out and full in front, so that when viewed from the side your chest will be thicker from front to back than your waist is. And at present, as you must realize, you are very little bigger around the chest than you are around the waist. Of course, your neck will get bigger as your chest gets bigger and your shoulders will get broader. You would look odd if you got a bigger chest and still had that slender neck. When I am through with you, you may have to wear a lS^-indh collar instead of that 13y₂ size you now have on. However, your neck will not look extra big, but in proportion to the rest of you."

It was no use! My neck had scared him off— which was a rather odd experience for me, as I had worked hard to develop my neck to its present size and shape. If I had talked all day I could not have made an impression on that man's mind. I felt just like a shoemaker does, when, after measuring a fat lady's foot and producing the right size shoe—five C—she insists that he does not know his business, and that in all her life she has never worn anything larger than a 2 double A; and if he cannot fit her there are other shoemakers, etc., etc.

Fashions and tastes change from year to year, but the ideal human figure does not. A beautifully made Greek athlete of 600 B.C. would be a beautifully made man of today. Conversely, a modern man, who wishes to make his body perfectly proportioned and supremely strong and enduring, cannot do better than to try and equal the proportions of some statue of Apollo, of Mercury, Theseus, Perseus, or one of the other old Greek heroes. There were well- built men before the time of the Greeks and there have been others since—even today.

I remember that when I was a boy the fashion in men's clothes was for the shoulders to be padded. Every man, in that year, who bought a new suit, immediately looked impossibly broad-shouldered. Sometimes there were pads as big as flat-irons where there should have been deltoid muscles. There was a great deal of talk about the "impressiveness of broad shoulders," and the "manly appearance of the new style." And since, like all boys, I aped my elders, I longed for the time when I could have one of those padded coats, and would be able to flaunt my (artificial) shoulders in the eyes of all beholders. Imagine my disgust when a couple of years later, I tried to get a coat of that variety, and the tailor said, "Oh I We are not padding the shoulders this year. The natural sloping shoulder is the thing."

A really well-made man does not have to depend on the cut of his clothes to give the impression of shapeliness. If he has the shape, the natural lines of his figure will set off any of the changing styles. This may sound more like a fashion-talk than a discussion of "the secrets of strength," but really it is important; because strength depends, as I hope to convince you, on the proportions of the body and on the size and quality of the muscles.

My hardest work is to convince a certain class of people that in order to become stronger and in general more vital, it is necessary to make themselves bigger. A man will tell me that he is tired of being a weakling, and would like to double or even triple his strength, if I can guarantee to do it in, say, six months. If, in reply, I say "Well, you have a good chance. I believe I can put six inches more around your chest, increase that 18-inch arm until it measures 15 inches, and give you a real pair of legs," he is apt to reply, "Oh! I don't want so much to be big-ger, as to be stronger " I can realize that if a rather tall man of thirty, has for ten years been wearing a 36 coat, it is somewhat of a shock to realize that in a few months he will have to be wearing a size 42; but when I show that man pictures of beautifully shaped modern athletes of his height, whose bodies have beautifully smooth lines, betokening both strength and agility; and tell him that their chests measure even more than 42 inches, he realizes that a large chest is necessary, and when it begins to dawn on him that instead of having to be apologetic about his slender arms, he will get an arm like a Dempsey or Sandow, he sees that after all there is some connection between vigor and proportions.

I suppose that a watchmaker gets used to the fact that a business man will carry a watch in his pocket for a life-time without having the least idea of how the watch works. But I cannot see how some young men, especially those interested in athletics, can live with their own bodies, and have so little knowledge of what their bodies should look like, and can be made to look like.

I found a young friend reading a book and he said, "Here is something that ought to interest you." I looked at the book, which told about Rajah Brooke's invasion of Borneo; and the paragraph started, "His crew were sturdy English fighting sailors—powerful men—not one of whom had less than a 14%-inch biceps." My friend said, "Say, Earle, is that a big arm?" I told him it was bigger than the average; such an arm as a blacksmith, a heavy-weight lifter or prizefighter might have—and that a $14^/2$ biceps might look very impressive on a short man, would seem inadequate on a very tall and broad-shouldered man, but nevertheless was a considerably bigger arm than the average man carried in his sleeve. Then, "Well, what is a really big arm," and I said, "Oh, sixteen to seventeen and a half inches according to the man's height."

Next, "How much does your arm measure?" I told him, and countered with, "And how about yours?" That struck home. He did not know his upper arm measurement, although he did know the measurement of his chest and waist because he ordered his own clothes; and he knew the size shoe and collar he wore. I suppose those things, together with his height and weight, are as much as the aver- age young fellow knows about his own body. But that the chest must be so many inches larger than the waist in order to give the proper taper to the body; that the chest itself must be of a certain size to insure proper lung capacity, and that a certain size arm should go with a certain size chest, is something of which even the athletically inclined are usually ignorant.

So when a man asks me to make him very much stronger without making him any bigger, I have to explain that I have no secret receptacle from which I can take a quantity of strength and pour it into his body. And even if I had, how could I put, say, a quart of strength into a vessel built to hold only a pint?

To put it in another way—you can't get eighty horse-power out of an engine which is built to develop only 40 H.P., no matter how much gas you feed into it. Even though it is true that it is the gas that makes the engine go, yet as a general rule the more the horse-power the bigger and finer the engine. And you simply cannot carry a five-ton load on a chassis built to carry tons as the limit.

There are "Strong Men" galore, and I defy you to bring me one who is either small, or weak looking. Oh! I know there are people—men and women both —who call themselves "Human Magnets"; who are frail in build, and who seem to do great feats of strength. But if you knew as much as I do about the show business, you would realize that these people's strength is literally an illusion.

Well then — among strong men we find chaps with 48-inch chests, with 17-inch arms, and 25-inch thighs. Some of them are lazy, and have allowed themselves to get fat and "beefy looking." But you can rest assured that, if they are the genuine article, underneath the fat you can see, there are hidden steel-like muscles. Most of them, however, "look the part"; and take pride in so doing. Their broad shoulders, deep chests, wide backs and muscular arms and legs all fit into the picture. And some of the biggest of them look amazingly slender. That is because they are big and strong in the right places. They have the size and development that gives enormous strength, and yet you can tell by looking at them, that they have not sacrificed one bit of their agility; nor does their imposing size make them clumsy. Because their development is rightly placed, it accentuates the beautiful lines of the figure. Positively one can become strong and powerfully built without making oneself, either very heavy, or in the least clumsy. I know two men of exactly the same height, one of whom is a professional "Strong Man" and the other is his manager. Both are big. Each is five feet, nine inches tall; but the manager has only a 40-inch chest and 14-inch arms; and is fat and has a 44-inch waist and weighs 220 pounds. While the athlete, who has a 44-inch chest, 16-inch arms, and a 32-inch waist, weighs 180 pounds. His hips are smaller because they carry no fat, but his legs are as big, far better shaped, and infinitely stronger than those of his manager. And he weighs forty pounds less, although he is a bigger framed man. True, he carries no fat except that small quantity which every healthy human being has to have. The bones of the two men are about the same size. If you could in any way segregate the pure muscular fiber of the fat manager, you would find that his actual muscles were only about half the size of the strong man's. All of which seems to prove that healthy well-trained muscular fiber weighs less than fat. It would be interesting to know just how much soft, useless fat a stout man carries around the middle of his body.

It is my experience that a man who is naturally slender, can so develop his body that it will be almost perfectly shaped; can increase his strength twofold or threefold, without the slightest danger of putting himself in the "truck-horse" class.

Let us take as an example, the average young fellow, say 23 or 24 years old. The likelihood is that he will stand about 5 feet 7% inches in height (for that is the average height), will weigh between 135 or 140 pounds clothed; and that he will take a "size 36" coat and a 14% collar. Now, if we make that man strip for a physical examination, we will find that by shedding his clothes his weight comes down close to 130 pounds. That removing his shoes has reduced his height to 5 feet 7 inches, or less. And his chest which he fondly imagines measures 36 inches because his coat is that size, actually measures between 34 and 35 inches. If you attire him in a pair of trunks and take his photograph, he is apt to be surprised and dismayed when he sees the picture. "Why" he will say "I had no idea I was so skinny as that. I look as though I could stand 20 pounds more weight." And it would be easy for him to put on that much weight simply by developing his muscles through the right kind of exercise.

The picture shows that he has just about as little muscular tissue as will enable his body and limbs to function. His back is about the same width all the way from shoulders to hips; almost without shape at all, and decidedly without that magnificent taper from arm-pits to waist that is shown by the really strong. The front of his body is perfectly smooth. His collar-bones which should be completely hidden, stick out like two rails. There is hardly an indication of the big muscles that should cover the chest, and his abdomen is as smooth and muscleless as that of a ten-year-old boy. Because he has always worn stiff collars, his neck is thin and pokes forward. His shoulder-blades protrude a bit. His arms measure perhaps about ten inches just below the elbow, and even less than that above the elbow, when the arms are hanging at the sides. His legs, which he has had to use in walking, are better than the rest of him; but the chances are that around the calves he measures not more than 13% inches, and that his thighs, even at the biggest part, measure 20 inches or less. Assuming that his work has been of a sedentary character, it is no wonder that his physique is so poor. The muscles grow by use, and the indoor workers—office men, clerks, students, and the like —hardly use their muscles at all. They are in the habit of riding even if they have only a few blocks to go; and during the day the hardest work they do is to pick up a ledger or move some light packages. Put such a fellow as I have described on a farm and you will almost see him grow from week-end to week-end. Because he is continually moving about —stooping, lifting, carrying, hoeing and pitching hay—he has to use almost all his muscles. His back will become thicker and broader; his shoulders will straighten up and get square in outline. His chest will be bigger. His legs in particular will get more sturdy and his arms will have a capable, sinewy look. In ten weeks of such outdoor work a young man will gain 20 pounds in weight; practically all of which is good solid muscle tissue. Naturally his eating has had something to do with it. Being continually in the open air in itself promotes appetite; but using his muscles ten hours a day is the real factor. For all that time he is putting forth energy and he will have to eat very much more in order to keep up his strength, than he did when working indoors. He sleeps soundly because he is healthily tired; he eats all he can get, and he is using his muscles practically all the time; and muscles grow from use. His gain in weight is due entirely to something new that he has created for himself—bigger muscles for the harder work.

You may tell me that all this is nothing new; that "Anybody knows that" When you go on a vacation and play games, or when you take a job at laboring, you expect to build up, and put on flesh if you are thin; and to reduce weight if you are fat. That you think, is the regular and natural thing.

Well, then, let us look at it from another angle. Grant that, at the end of your ten weeks on the farm, you are a huskier physical specimen than when you started in. You look better, you feel better, and you know you are better. You can carry a heavy sack of potatoes that you could not have even lifted on the first day; you can keep on for hours at back-breaking labor that would have crippled you in the old days. You have a grand feeling of hardiness and capability. (And all of that is the result of im-systematic work, that is, unsystematic muscular work. For farm labor, while it calls heavily on certain muscles, leaves others almost untouched.) When you look at yourself in a mirror, you seem to be bigger all around than previously; but except in a few places there are but few indications of any pronounced increase in the size and shape of the muscles. Your back is infinitely better, for you have somehow acquired two big cables of muscle along each side of the spine, and there seems to be two or three times as much muscle across your shoulder blades as before. The points of your shoulders are much rounder. Your forearms are perhaps an inch bigger, your hands bigger and harder, and even your wrists seem thicker. Your thighs while not so very much bigger, are rounder than formerly, and look bigger when you view them from the side. All that is gratifying, but you are somewhat puzzled by the fact that your upper arms have not become as big and round and heavily muscled as the rest of you. You have developed but little muscle on the front of the body itself (breast and abdomen) and the front and sides of the thighs have not assumed those big, swelling, and impressive curves you are accustomed to see on the legs of track athletes, football players and tumblers.

But that you have gained at all is gratifying, and you feel if you could afford it you would always do several hours' muscular work every day. If you did, you would in all probability be disappointed in the results. For after a very few months of daily hard labor you would find that the body would lose its power to more than renew itself. That the work instead of steadily increasing your size and strength, would tend to tire you; that your energy would gradually be drained, and that instead of having a surplus you would have a deficit.

Laboring men and farmers are undoubtedly, as a class, stronger than indoor workers; but also, as a class, they are not very strong. No laborer uses his back more than a coal-heaver, yet the average oarsman who rows only a hundred hours in the whole year, is apt to have a stronger back than the average coal-heaver. Similarly a gymnast who uses his arm muscle only an hour a day will have a stronger arm than the average blacksmith who uses his arm eight times as much. I can use this undoubted fact to prove to you that it takes very much less time and trouble to develop a strong body than it does to properly train your mind, and that systematic exercise produces more strength than does hard labor.

Because I have always been interested in muscular development, I am a close observer of the effects of different kinds of exercise, and different schemes of training. Arid always I have found that methodical, svstematic exercise produces vastly greater results in muscle making and strength building than does, hit-or-miss unsystematic work.

We have seen how a slender young fellow can add considerably to his bodily weight and muscular strength by getting outdoors and doing actual labor. As far as general improvement is concerned, he can get just about as much net results by working in a gymnasium for an hour each evening, during ten successive weeks. I say "working" advisedly; because I believe that it is impossible to get a high degree of either muscle, or strength, unless you work for it. If you join a "gymnasium class" and spend the whole session in performing elementary drills, such as waving the arms, and gently bending the body this way and that, you will, to be sure, awaken your muscular system and improve your circulation, but you will not gain perceptibly in development; nor will you become very much stronger. If, however, you go to a "gym" which is not given up entirely to "class-work," which is patronized by men who like "real exercise," and where you have the unrestricted use of all the apparatus, you can increase the size and strength of your muscles just as much or more, than you can by outdoor labor.

Suppose after a week or two spent at doing easy stunts, your muscles commence to harden up, and you attempt the more vigorous stunts that give them harder and harder work. At the end of the month or so when you go to the gym, instead of spending the hour doing mild calisthenics your program is something like this: You get on the flying rings and do a few stunts to limber yourself up. You practice a bit at bar-vaulting, raising the bar after each vault. You join some of the other members and practice some tumbling and hand-balancing stunts. You do some rope climbing, "chinning the bar," "dipping" on the parallels; pull away vigorously for a few minutes on the rowing-machine; use the springboard for your legs and the "rack" for your abdominal and side muscles; and maybe wind up the evening at a bout of wrestling with some active opponent.

Under such a program you can, and will build up rapidly. Just as rapidly as though you spent all your waking hours at labor. You exercise pretty much all of your muscles, and because you do things which require strength, you create the strength with which to do them. And at the end of a few weeks you will find that you have outgrown your clothes, and that your friends are remarking at your improved appearance.

The effects of this kind of gym work are more visible than the effects of farm work, and also of a different character. While work on the farm provides active exercise, and increased strength in the back, the shoulders, the forearms and part of the legs; the gym work tends to give less work to those parts and more to the upper arms, the chest, and abdominal and side muscles, and to other, and different muscles on the legs. Moreover, gym work makes you springier and more active than does farm labor, produces almost as good an appetite and certainly makes your muscles stand out more prominently.

But even then, such unsystematic gym practice does not create great strength; all it does is to make you as strong as the others who use the gym. And while the average all-round gymnast is stronger than the average farmer, or day laborer, and very much stronger and better developed than the average man; yet he falls far short of being as strong as those men who have deliberately trained with the idea of becoming as strong and as well-shaped as is possible for a man to be.

In the course of a day's work the farm-hand may have to exert the full strength of his back muscles only once or twice. In the course of an evening's workout, the gymnast may do many things which require a full and powerful contraction of his muscles. Which explains why the gymnast's arm muscles, for instance, are bigger, better-developed, and more powerful than those of the farm-hand. It is a truism to say that the strongest muscle is the one which can contract against the greatest resistance; but it is not generally known that the contractile strength of a muscle can be purposely and definitely increased by training it to contract against an ever-increasing resistance. The same power can be developed by causing the muscles to make what is known as a "full contraction" instead of the partial contraction which is all that is required when working or doing gymnastic stunts.

Anyone who has spent much of his time around gymnasiums is familiar with the remarkable development that comes from specializing in certain kinds of vigorous work, and the incredible strength which comes from such development. I was only a kid when I first joined a gym, and more by good luck than by good management, I happened to pick out one that was patronized by a lot of professional athletes, gymnasts and stage performers. Everything, in fact, from contortionists to circus "Strong Men."

Each of these men was in his way a specialist who earned his living by his trained muscles; and since I associated with them daily and watched them train, I naturally learned a lot.

I would watch a jumper training his thigh muscles and a gymnast coaxing up his arm strength. I recall there were two men in that crowd who particularly aroused my enthusiasm. One of them was a "Roman Ring Artist" who was at that time a great drawing-card in the big vaudeville circuits. The extraordinary thing about him was his arm and shoulder development. Up to then I had never seen such arms. I never thought to ask him how much they measured, but I suppose they must have spanned close to 17 inches. Even when he walked around, just swinging his arms naturally, the biceps and triceps muscles between the elbow and shoulder would ripple and roll under the skin in a way that fascinated me. And his shoulders! Well, he was not particularly broad, but covering the points of the shoulders were deltoid muscles literally as big as cocoanuts. His breast-muscles were as big as any I have ever seen, and his back seemed like a mass of interwoven straps, and ropes of muscle.

Every day when he came in for practice, he would walk over to the rings, pull himself up very slowly, shift his weight from one hand to the other, curl with one hand at a time, do "Planches" and other revolutions; but always very, very slowly.

When I asked him why he always started off with these slow movements, he told me that it was because it was much harder to do the things slowly, and required more strength. That he had to have a lot of strength, for that when he did his stuff before an audience it was necessary to do the hardest tricks as though they were easy to him. He also explained to me the necessity of fully flexing the muscles and told me how he had "worked up" his strength. Like most specialists he had an uneven development. He had the torso and arms of a Hercules, and the legs and hips of a non-athletic person. See him only from the waist up and you would guess that he weighed 180 pounds. See only his legs and he looked like a 125-pounder. So he must originally have had a small frame, and it would be interesting to know whether he could have developed legs equally as good as his arms if he had trained his leg muscles as thoroughly as he had his arms. Then he was very strong in certain ways but not in others. He could tear three packs of cards, and it was a cinch for him to twist iron bars in the way that at present seems so wonderful to some of you. I doubt though, whether he could have lifted a very heavy weight off the ground, simply because he didn't have the legs for that kind of stunt; and I imagine that he could not have carried 500 pounds on one shoulder the way that some "Strong Men" carry twice that much. Because, in the first place, the muscles at the sides of his waist were not strong enough to keep him from doubling over sideways, and in the second place his legs were so frail that they would have buckled at the knees at the first step.

Undoubtedly he was a strong-armed man, but whether he was a "Strong Man" is a question, for no man is really strong unless he is strong all over.

Another man in that gym, who interested me, was an old gentleman who was one of the few amateurs who frequented the place. I did not know his exact age, but from things he said I judged that he was a boy in Civil War days, and must have become interested in exercise in the 1870's; a time at which there was a vogue for a device called a "health-lift." All he was interested in was lifting weights off the floor; and he had made a contraption on which he could load a 100-pound weight and at the top of the affair was a handle, or cross-bar, which reached up about twenty-eight inches. This man had the theory that if every day you thoroughly exercised your back muscles, you would keep your figure, your health, and your strength into advanced old age. So every afternoon he would drop in and have a short session with his lifting-machine. He would pile on three or four hundred pounds, stand with straight legs, bend his body by arching his spine a trifle, and lift the weight by straightening his back. He would put on more weights and practice what professionals call the "hand-and-thigh" lift. He would keep his back straight and bend his legs at the knees, grasp the handle-bar, so that his knuckles would rest against the front of the thigh; and lift the weight by straightening the legs and heaving up the shoulders. After two or three repetitions he would pile on more weight, and it was customary to work up to 1,000 or 1,200 pounds before he quit. On one occasion to settle an argument he lifted 1,500 pounds dead weight in the £"hand-and-thigh style." I cannot tell you how long he had exercised in that way, but he must have been at it forty years when I knew him. And as he rarely missed a day, there was very good reason for his profound faith in his own method of keeping himself strong and healthy. As a result of his specialized work he had a most peculiar development. His thighs, both back and front, were unusually big and his calves were enormous. Naturally he had big chains of muscles along the spine, but the striking thing was the phenomenal development of the trapezius muscles, which are in the upper back just below the base of the neck. These muscles, when they contract, "shrug up" the shoulders, and when he did his "hand-and-thigh" lift and heaved his shoulders up, you could see these muscles bunch themselves into two enormous masses. Even when standing at ease these muscles were so big that they made his shoulders slope at a high angle up from the deltoids to the sides of his neck. No ready-made coat would fit him. His forearms—especially the outside parts of them—were covered with muscles so powerfully developed that there were big furrows between them. His grip was something to be avoided. His biceps muscles were pronounced in their size, but his whole upper arm was small compared to his forearm; and notwithstanding his ability to lift enormous weights from the ground he could not lift big dumb-bells over head. My objections to his plan were, that by giving very heavy work to only a few sets of muscles he had made those muscles stiff and rather slow in action; and by his specialization he had failed both to realize the full strength of his whole body and had spoiled the symmetry of that body.

I was particularly interested in the effects of his exercise. So far as I could see, his heart was perfectly sound and strong, and as an explanation he told me that he never lifted so much that it made him red in the face. The moment he felt that there was a strain on the blood-vessels, he would stop and lighten the weight. You might think that his constant dead-weight lifting would have broken down the arches in his feet, but the exact opposite was the case, for the work which developed the big muscles in his calves seemed to give equal strength to the muscles of the feet.

Then there was the man who used nothing but pulley-weights. Nowadays the pulley-weights you find in gymnasiums are small things, equipped with a few weights of a pound apiece. But this one was a massive affair with thick cords and provided with ten weights of five pounds each. So, if you cared to, you could put 25 pounds on the end of each pulley. This enthusiast never stood up when exercising, because, he said, when you stood on your feet you unconsciously used your body weight to help in the work. So he would sit on a stool facing the pulley weights; and would go through a lot of movements very slowly and steadily. Then he would reverse, and sit with his back to the machine and do a lot more. I have seen him work for thirty minutes without stopping and at the end of that time the surrounding floor would be wet with his sweat. Certainly he had a wonderful development from the diaphragm upwards, but below the level of his lowest ribs he was only average.

In those days they cared for nothing except big arm, shoulder and upper-body development. If they had their pictures taken they knew but one pose, and that was to sit in a chair with their arms folded across the chest and the biceps muscles pushed out by the hidden fingers.

There was a man who pinned all his faith to the "upright parallels"—a pair of bars set perpendicular to the floor instead of horizontal. The thing was to stand between these bars, grasp one in each hand at the height of your nipples, and then to lunge the body forwards and backwards. According to this man that was the only exercise anyone needed. "For," he said, "when you throw your weight backwards you develop all the muscles on the rear half of your body, and also strengthen your back, and when you lunge forward and through the bars, you open up the chest and develop all the muscles on the front of your body. If you don't believe it look at me." And that would end the argument, for when you looked him over you could not but admit the beauty of his build. None of these muscles were very big, but they were all good-sized. His chest was roomy and he had, I think, the widest back I have ever seen on a man of his height. The general lines of his figure were grand. He gave credit to the upright parallels for all his development— even for his fine legs. It happened that three or four times a week he would play handball for one hour, and he apparently forgot that that was what developed his legs—for the upright parallels positively will not make the legs either much bigger or much stronger.

Looking back I can see where I must have been an awful nuisance to some of those men, for I was continually pestering them with questions and trying to drag information out of them. I fear I have always been that way. If I saw a man with amazing muscles in his chest I would have to know what he did to develop them. If a man had large and wonderfully shaped thighs I would ask him how they got that way; and whether the legs just grew that way, or whether he had succeeded in giving them their size and shape by exercising; and if so, what exercises did he favor. I was a "bear" on measurements and would embarrass these athletes by demanding to know exactly how much—to a fraction of an inch—their arms, legs and chests measured.

I may have been over-zealous, but I sure learned a lot. I found that the better a man was, the more willing he was to help you. After all, the secrets of acquiring strength are: first, to know what to do, and second, to do it. So these wise old birds had no hesitation in telling me just how to improve my development, and increase my strength, because they knew very well that it would not help me unless I had the ambition to become strong and the willingness to work to get strong. Today people consider that I am exceptionally well developed—all I can say is that I deserve to be, because I certainly worked for it.

39

www.ingramcontent.com/pod-product-compliance
Lightning Source LLC
Chambersburg PA
CBHW070239290526
45789CB00004B/1694